YOUR JOURNEY TOWARDS FERTILITY

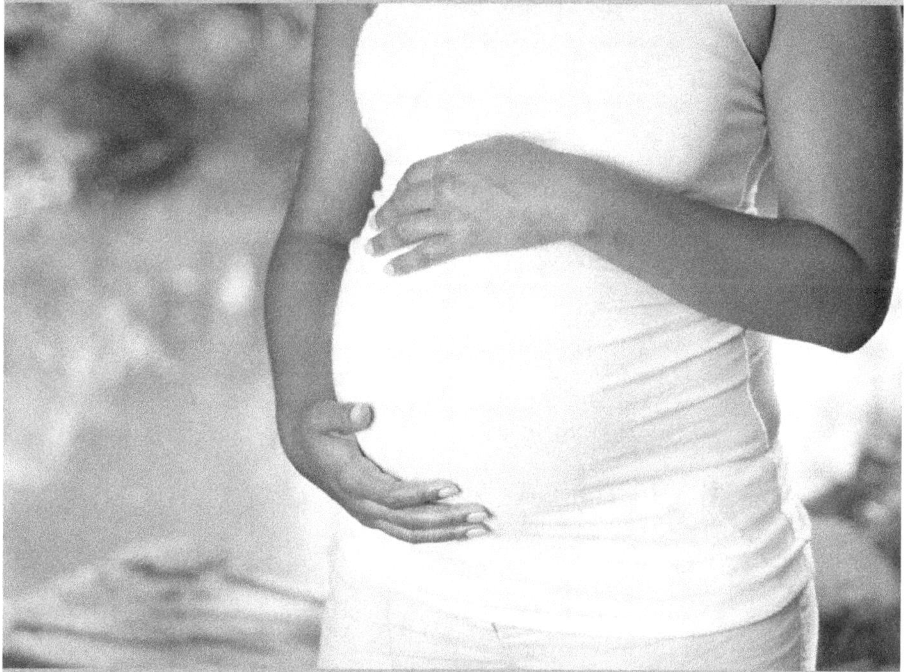

Spiritual Dimensions

Janice N. Njie

YOUR JOURNEY TOWARDS FERTILITY

Spiritual Dimensions

Janice N. Njie

This book is essentially written in British English. How-ever, other variations of the English language, mostly the American English, are used in order to preserve the origin-ality of most of the works quoted here which were writ-ten in other English variants.

ISBN: 9798691828096

Email: aterejanice@yahoo.com;
janicenjie73@gmail.com

ABOUT THE BOOK

This book was birth in the course of helping women to spiritually deal with their challenge of infertility. It is also a call to share the story of my fertility journey with other women and help them find some encouragement and courage in the face of their own struggles.

Fertility is not just a matter of biological science. It is a spiritual journey involving the fulfillment of one of our creator's design for our lives as human beings and as a race. Therefore our arch enemy the devil is deeply interested in how, why and when we procreate as human beings. There will always be some scientific explanations as to the whys certain things happen in our lives. However, we all know that our human science at its best has numerous limitations and a lot is still left to guess work while researches are ongoing. Humans will always be used for experimentations in one way or the other. When it comes to the issue of infertility, a lot is left to the unknown. Even at its best, fertility medicine has a huge chasm of unanswered questions. It is said that the science can answer questions from when and how eggs and sperms are produced, how fertilization takes place, and so on. But the science still cannot fully explain the miracle of conception. The two weeks after Embryo transfer (implantation period) in fertility treatment will always be left to the unknown and shrouded in mystery.

The war over the continuity and sustenance of the human race is a very fierce one. And the devil is doing all he can, using every possible means to interfere with how humans obey the divine mandate of procreation.

As human beings, we must begin to ask critical questions before adopting everything offered to us in the name of scientific solutions. We must adopt some scientific protocols with a "pinch of salt" like the saying goes.

When we begin to hear statements like "population control" we should be careful. Population control is not the same thing as family planning. Family planning is the sugar coating of something deeper and bigger.

If you aim at reducing the population of a particular place by all means, it also means you are increasing the human population of another place. And where is that Hell. Depopulate earth and populate hell.

The chain of negative events that usually follow couples dealing with infertility is an endless list. From adulteries, bitterness, hatred, divorces, trauma, murder, we can go on and on.

My prayer is that we will begin to look beyond the natural and also see the supernatural /spiritual dimensions attached to the battle over human procreation. And therefore as we pursue the various options as solutions, we bring in the God factor that always makes the ultimate difference in our quest for fertility health.

God bless you!

DEDICATION

This book is dedicated to every family on Earth dealing with the challenge of Infertility.

CHAPTER ONE

1.1. Introduction

We will be writing from the perspective that as tripartite beings we as humans were created as spirits, living in a body, possessing a soul. Therefore whenever there is discord in any aspect of our nature as humans, our whole being will be affected one way or the other.

For the continuity of our race, we were created as a combination of spiritual, social as well as sexual beings. With the ability to derive pleasure from our sexuality and procreate through it. Therefore any distortion in the way we handle our sexuality, be it in our mindset or spirit will translate into our bodies affecting our overall well-being. With presentations of all kinds of diseases including infertility and mental disorder.

Everything is connected. You cannot dissociate spiritual/emotional wellness from physical wellness and vice versa. And when it comes to fertility, the stakes gets higher and very glaring because it becomes a social, cultural, religious, and global issue as well.

We said before that the Bible is our premise and foundation for spiritual wellness. Many have scorned basic life principles written in the Bible to their own ruin. In the Book also lie answers to some very pressing life and global issues. But the Book is coded as if it were. Only true God seekers will find their answers. A critical and high minded spirit will find the Bible very antagonistic and thus it will become a stumbling block. Because it will only be seen as a Book that wants to stop humans from enjoying their lives.

However, The Creator wants us all to live very fulfilled and healthy lives. His command and His desire for us is that we should be productive in every sphere of our lives. To enjoy all the good things that life has to offer. But things changed. And now, we have so many distortions, aberrations, deviations and perversions to deal with. And all around us, we see humanity and the whole of creation in distress. The Bible calls it groaning. Creation is groaning in pain and agony.

1.2. Scientific Overview of Infertility

Infertility is typically defined as the inability to achieve pregnancy after one year of unprotected intercourse. If you have been trying to conceive for a year or more, you should consider an infertility evaluation. However, if you are 35 years or older, you should consider beginning the infertility evaluation after about six months of unprotected intercourse rather than a year.

- Infertility affects an estimated 15% of couples globally, amounting to 48.5 million couples.
- Males are found to be solely responsible for 20-30% of infertility cases and contribute to 50% of cases overall.

(Agarwal A, Mulgund A, Hamada A, Chyatte MR. A unique view on male infertility around the globe. Reprod Biol Endocrinol. 2015;13:37. Published 2015 Apr 26. doi:10.1186/s12958-015-0032-1)

Frequent intercourse without birth control usually results in pregnancy:

- For 50% of couples within 3 months
- For 75% within 6 months
- For 90% within 1 year

1.3. Definition
Infertility is usually defined as the inability of a couple to achieve a pregnancy after repeated intercourse without contraception

for 1 year.

1.4. Causes of Infertility

- The cause of infertility may be due to problems in the man, the woman, or both:
- Problems with sperm (in 35% or more of couples)
- Problems with ovulation (in about 20%)
- Problems with the fallopian tubes and abnormalities in the pelvis (in about 30%)
- Problems with cervical mucus (in 5% or fewer)
- Unidentified factors (in about 10%)
- Unhealthy lifestyle options like, tobacco smoking, recreational drugs, poor diet, excessive exercise, excess caffeine.

1.5. Diagnosis

The diagnosis of infertility problems requires a thorough assessment of both partners. Usually, the assessment is done after at least 1 year of trying to achieve a pregnancy.

1.6. When to Seek Help for Infertility

- The woman is over 35 (usually after 6 months of trying to become pregnant).
- The woman's menstrual periods occur infrequently (fewer than nine a year).
- The woman has a previously identified abnormality of the uterus, fallopian tubes, or ovaries.
- Doctors have identified or suspect problems with sperm in the man.
- Age is a factor, especially for women. As women age, becoming pregnant becomes more difficult, and the risk of complications during pregnancy increases.

- Also, women, particularly after age 35, have a limited time to resolve infertility problems before menopause.

1.7. Treatment

- Treatment depends on the cause of infertility.
- It involves the use of medications to treat hormonal imbalances, treat infections, induce ovulation (like in the cases of ovarian disorders, or sperm disorders), surgery to correct organ dysfunction, malformations, or blockages.
- Assisted reproductive therapies.
- Measures to lessen stress, including counseling and other forms of holistic support.

1.8. The Goals of Treatment Are

- To treat the cause of infertility if possible
- To make conception more likely
- To reduce the time needed to conceive

1.9. Prevention

- Properly treat every form of sexually transmitted disease
- Healthy lifestyles
- Avoid the use of untested concoctions to treat suspected infertility at home.
- Visit a fertility expert in for your fertility needs.

CHAPTER 2

2.1. Fertility Beyond Science

Ex 23:26; and none will miscarry or be barren in your land. I will give you a full life span. (NIV)
John 10:10: I am come that they might have life, and that they might have it more abundantly (KJV)

If humanity explains everything that happens in life and in our world simply on the basis of science, then we will be missing out on other key solutions to human problems and challenges. As beings, we are created as compound beings with spirit soul and a body. Most times our physical well-being is the last part of us that shows that there is some chaos going on. The key part of our person that plays a role in our overall well-being is our spirits and our mindset.

And our base book which is the Bible tells us to guard our hearts because out of it comes issues of life. A healthy spiritual and mental state will mean that we will do everything it takes to ensure that our overall choices enhances wholesomeness and wellness.

But because we have consistently pushed or numb the most sensitive part of our being, we have allowed into our global spaces factors that works against our very essence. Factors that have negatively impacted our core self. The more advancement humanity makes in science and technology, the more complex and complicated life become. So it is no longer our individual choices that are hostile to our ability to fulfill our mandate of procreation, but the overall choices of some who have delegated themselves as custodians of planet Earth with the responsibility of managing global population by all means. Including decided who, why, when and we should procreate.

So with increase scientific advancement comes increase in what I call the **"Death Seals."**Things that carry with it the tinge of **death** as it's after math. Death trails every major scientific development. You can name it from medical, to automobile, aeronautics, agricultural, entertainment, media technologies. Most times their effect on human reproduction is gross. But because it's a vicious circle, we produce antidotes and come up with ways to mitigate the negative effects of our own very technological advancements. Thus we have for the management of the inability to procreate, Assisted Reproductive Therapies (ART). Ways to help those who cannot reproduce through natural sexual activity can now do it asexually through ART. Great right? But still ART has it's gross limitations and is laden by many unanswered questions.

- ◦ Live Births per Egg Retrieval:
- ◦ For women younger than 35, the percentage of live births per egg retrieval is 54.4 percent.
- ◦ For women ages 35 to 37, the percentage of live births per egg retrieval is 42 percent.
- ◦ For women ages 38 to 40, the percentage of live births per egg retrieval is 26.6 percent.
- ◦ For women ages 41 to 42, the percentage of live births per egg retrieval is 13.3 percent.
- ◦ For women ages 43 and up, the percentage of live births per egg retrieval is 3.9 percent.

So we can see that there are still a lot of limitations. Even though things are getting "better."

2.2. Infertility Self Worth

In my two decades of career as a nurse even long before I started working with clients dealing with infertility, I came across many women who felt they were not complete simply because they were having issues conceiving. In some cases, their husbands had categorically rejected every attempt to go for medical checkup so that they can together make informed decisions on how to handle their challenge. Prior to when both couples faces the storm together, the woman lives with the full weight of the issue of childlessness in their family. In our African cultural context, she is stigmatized, maligned and sometimes insulted publicly even by other women.

I got pregnant after eight years with my son's father at the age of 36. But throughout that period, I never missed my night's sleep because of the issue. And I didn't give anyone permission to maltreat me because of the fact that I have not had a child. I told the only person who felt he had the right to rebuke me about the fact that I had not brought forth a son into the family that, if he were to be a god I would have knelt down and prayed to him for the fruit of the womb. But if he isn't a god and cannot join me in praying for the fruit of the womb, then he should never harass me again! He was so shocked that he simply walked away from me. And that was the end of discussion.

As women, we are creatures of enormous potentials. If one of your assets has been touched concentrate on what is working instead of burying everything else on the altar of childlessness. Most women and couples build a monument around their challenge of child birth and start worshiping it. That monument determines how they interact and interpret everything else. It becomes a magnifying glass that determines not only how they interpret others, but also how they see themselves. The monument's overflow with toxic emotions of bitterness, self doubts, jealousy, guilt(especially for women who have had abortions),hatred, malice, self pity, anger, self preservation, and many other such negative emotions. The cultivation of these emotions creates an atmosphere that works against their very desire for conception. Because nothing really grows or thrives on toxic soil. We do not have control over how people treat us. But we have complete control how we respond. And that also depends on how we see ourselves. If you start seeing yourself as a failure and a half creature simply because you are dealing with the challenge of infertility, people will automatically start seeing you that way and treating you in like manner.

When God created us all, He also prepared all the resources we will need to fulfill His purposes for our lives. But the world is like a garden of roses. Hidden between the beautiful rose flowers are thorns and thistles. It is a battle field. We can only navigate our way through looking at the One who holds the compass. Jesus Christ. Not sciences, not our status, our culture, our wealth, our education and so forth. None of those things can offer us permanent solutions to our life's challenges. Only God can if we go to him. You would tell me that many people are praying for the fruit of the womb and yet they are not getting answers. How do they plan to receive answers with hearts filled up with negative emotions and vibrations? The Bible says the gifts God gives addeth no sorrows. Some have gone to the devil himself to transact and exchange that will eventually make them conceive.

Sadly most times it happens just close to their break through and the devil perpetually holds them hostage over his "gift." A gift that always comes with untold sorrows. I told someone once that if anyone is to feel shame for your childlessness it would be God. But He is not moved because He has already answered your prayer before you ever asked. None was created barren. We were all created with the ability to carry our own babies. So what are the issues?

It is therefore, very important to uproot from your mind every thought that contradicts conception. Thoughts and feelings of unworthiness, guilt and fear and so on. We will be handling that during the prayer session. By decreeing God's word concerning you as far as fertility is concerned.

2.3. To Each His Own Battle

There is no human being on this earth who is not dealing with a challenge. We are on a battle field. Some are dealing with untold hardship, some with chronic diseases, other with gross poverty, some with blindness, deafness, deformities, others with addictions, obsessions, pervasive behaviors and so on and so forth. Some have multiple problems others just a few. But each person feels that theirs is the biggest issue. So it is important not to be absorbed with your own problems to the point that you do not see anything else. I once met a woman in the fertility clinic where I worked sometime ago. Once she enters the clinic, I could practically touch her bitterness and anger. She comes in ready to fight. Like a wounded lion. My boss asked me if I can work with people who are wounded. I told him I worked with some of the most sensitive cases in medical history and my gifts of healing comes in to play in all the complicated situations I face. I always aim for spiritual and emotional healing. Once that is attained the rest is easy. The science of the drugs can easily be managed. But the inwards bruises are the most sensitive part. God always picks out some people and tells me how to minister to them. In this particular case, the Lord told me she will not be pregnant if she doesn't give up that bitterness. So once we were together, I asked her to let go of the pain the bitterness and the hurt that is eating her up. Told her it will affect her results. She told me I will not understand. I told her I did. It took me eight years into marriage to get pregnant. I was a missionary, no money for IVF even if it existed, nothing. I simply surrendered that part of my life to God and told Him it was his business to give me a child if I must have one. While I go about serving others as a missionary nurse. I received insults, was treated like a small secondary school girl by many. And yet, I refused to feed any negative emotions around that. I held her inside that small room, prayed for her as directed by the Lord. With my hands placed on her abdomen. Afterward, we handed the burden over to the Lord. She cast that care at the feet of the Lord. You could see an outward transformation come over her. I didn't know she was that pretty with a wonderful dimpled smile. I made her a promise to take her out for a treat even if she doesn't get pregnant. But reassured her if she leaves that burden to the One who holds the answer, she will celebrate in the end. She got pregnant. You can only imagine the rest of the story. She had done IVF more than five times. The Lord led me to minister to many like that. Most of whom got pregnant. Sometimes the Lord will simply ask me to lay hands on a woman and make declarations. Some were Christians, some were Muslims. On a few occasions, a woman would simply take my hands and place it on their abdomen asking me to pray for them. I would wait on the Lord for directions on how to minister to them. Other times the Lord will tell me this one will not be pregnant and explains why. In everything, I saw God's hand in the whole process. Sometimes on night duty, He will lead me to pray specific prayers for specific people. So my work had a lot to do with spiritual and emotional healing than just injecting these women with medications.

A lot of these women kept in touch even when I left. One particularly touching call was that of a woman who called thanking me. I thought she was pregnant. Only for her to tell me that it was the counseling sessions I had with her that gave her the courage to accept the results. She could handle the negative test results with hope.

I cried after that call. She surrendered her pain to the Lord. I know she will eventually get pregnant.

2.4. Toxic Spiritual and Emotional Environment

If you are in a toxic relationship or surrounded by toxic spiritual atmosphere, our first job is to eliminate the toxicity before conception. Otherwise you will carry and give birth to a child who will have to fight battles you created for them. So another thing to handle when preparing for conception is our environment. Creating an atmosphere that supports wholesomeness and wellness. Because babies in the womb have unadulterated sensitiv- ities to the environment around which they are being nurtured. I will leave it at that for now.

CHAPTER THREE

3.1. World Views

The universe has its order of things. Whenever anyone tampers with that order they face consequences. Just a matter of time. You cannot maltreat and emotionally traumatize another human being and go scot free. Doesn't matter how long it takes. You must and will pay. Any man or woman who torments another person for the challenges or trouble they might be going through, even if they brought it on themselves will suffer some consequences. Did God send you to help him punish another for their mistakes? I have heard women talk mockingly about the fact that so and so person is suffering because of the abortions they committed. Who appointed you judge? It is better to keep quiet if you do not have compassion to show. The God of mercy and compassion always knows when to step in to solve the problems of those who go to Him for solutions. I will end this here for now.

3.2. A Sure Promise

Ezekiel 12:28"Therefore say to them, 'This is what the Sovereign Lord says: None of my words will be delayed any longer; whatever I say will be fulfilled, declares the Sovereign Lord.'"
Philippians 1:6: being confident of this, that he who began a good work in you will carry it on to completion until the day of Christ Jesus.

Ecc 3:11He hath made everything beautiful in its time: also he hath set eternity in their heart, yet so that man cannot find out the work that God hath done from the beginning even to the end.

The song writer wrote "the things He has promised He will bring them to pass. By the Stripes that He bore, we have been healed.

Every promise of God in the Bible is Yea and Amen. It is sealed. But we need to lay hold of His promises from a point of faith. And not fear. Faith and fear are mutually exclusive. And most of us often times approach God's promises from the point of fear and helplessness. He delights in fulfilling His promises in our lives. Any one of God's promises that has not been made manifest in our lives is delaying either because it is not time for it's fulfillment or that we are approaching God not by faith but from a point of fear. That actually blocks His blessings.

3.3. Infertility from a Victory Stand

Infertility is not a death sentence. Some women think that it is children that keep a marriage. Companionship was the first reason why God decided to grant the man his heart's desire. The Bible says in;

Gen 2:20-23 20And Adam gave names to all cattle, and to the fowl of the air, and to every beast of the field; but for Adam there was not found an help meet for him.

21And the LORD God caused a deep sleep to fall upon Adam, and he slept: and he took one of his ribs, and closed up the flesh instead thereof; 22And the rib, which the LORD God had taken from man, made he a woman, and brought her unto the man.

23And Adam said, this is now bone of my bones, and

flesh of my flesh: she shall be called Woman, because she was taken out of Man.

He was still lonely even after naming all the other creatures. He wasn't thinking about someone to make babies with. He was looking for a companion to share his life and work with! He was not looking for a baby factory. He was looking for a companion.

Making babies was a part of God's Divine mandate to both of them. It wasn't the woman's responsibility to conjure pregnancy. Procreation was an assignment to the both of them. Both of them were to make it happen. The whole trauma poured on the woman for the production of children and in some cases; she is molested for not birthing male children is an aberration.

3.4. The Concept of Motherhood

Isaiah 54:1"Shout for joy, O barren woman, who bears no children; break forth into song and cry aloud, you who have never travailed; because more are the children of the desolate woman than of her who has a husband," says the LORD.
Psalm 113:9 He gives the childless woman a household, making her the joyful mother of children. Hallelujah!

I have heard many statements like your own is your own. Women, even when they get to the point when they realize that carrying a pregnancy may jeopardize their health still went ahead and got pregnant only to satisfy that thing they perceive is as being a complete woman. And a lot of them have lost their lives in the process.   I watched a video Yesterday of a young boy of about eight who was beaten or rather battered by the woman he calls his mother. I wept and felt so much pain. It was as if I could hear his innermost cry. Women getting married to men who already had kids and suffered from "Cinderella's step mother's syndrome."Maltreating their step children while praying for God to give them their own. Another woman did surrogacy and later got became pregnant. And started maltreating the children from the surrogate mother. What justifications do women have for maltreating other people's children? Sometimes it is the maid or the young boy from the village. Any woman who maltreats another woman's child is betraying the very essence of motherhood. Because motherhood talks of that intrinsic ability to nurture, groom another person to maturity and responsibility. And it has nothing to do with the ability to attain conception and giving birth to life babies. If that were to be the case, women will not be throwing their babies in rubbish dump, or burying them alive after carrying them for nine months.

So God has the ability to enable the Barren woman to nurture children and build her home. Psalm 113:9 and Isa 54: 1.

3.6. Factors Affecting Fertility

Factors affecting Fertility falls into three categories.

Physical factors that has to do with organ defects like polycystic ovaries, tubal blockages hormonal disorder for both male and females and Emotional/Psychological factors like trauma, toxics relationships, mindset and so on.

Spiritual Factors: Whereas physical factors are objective and can be treated with structured therapeutic protocols, spiritual factors are often times subjective even though they have the potential of causing great damages.

These can be as a result of unhealthy spiritual covenants, altars or yokes. In some cases the victim is aware. But in other instances the victims are not active participants but rather passive victims of the choices of usually parents or husbands. But it usually has to do with someone close enough to negotiate diabolic transactions that can affect a person through witchcraft and occultism.

Whatever it is, we also have a power that can counteract every form of transaction even the ones you did by yourself. Once you realize your error, acknowledge your sin and repent, you can annul anything else that does not tally with God's purposes for your life. And barrenness is not the will of God for anybody. There is no Scripture that says that God appointed some to be barren. Therefore you can annul every covenant, shatter every altar and break every yoke that does not conform to the will of God for your life.

Satan does not give free gifts. God is the only One who gives free gifts. So whenever an individual becomes desperate enough for something and goes to the devil, he must of necessity carry out an exchange.

I have had to minister to women and receive revelations of their fathers coming to them in a dream and asking for their eggs when they were kids. And as adults they come face to face with an inability to produce eggs. And therefore become pregnant. In one instance, I told a woman that if we pray for God to break whatever was done to obstruct fertility; it will affect the person who did the transaction. She then asked me to hold on. And narrated her dream as a young teenage girl who just started seeing her period. She said a few weeks after that dream, her dad suddenly but suspiciously hit jackpot! So she was afraid. She didn't want to hurt her dad. She loves him. Said her dad has been good to her. That he used the money well. And she is not that desperate to have a baby. She decided to go for surrogacy. Again the father refused. And told her there is no rush. Mind you she is above mid 50s. At that point, I rested my case. Right now she is working on possible adoption.

A woman held me one day in the office while I was on night duty, she had just finished her fertility procedure. She begged me to pray for her. Her husband was there. I coaxed her and went ahead and gave her injection. Thinking that by the time we finished, they will be in a hurry to leave since it was late in the night. But when she finished she waited for me. I sorted after the Lord and received go ahead to pray for her. As I was praying, there were so many demonic activities around her. Her husband who was sitting nonchalantly suddenly stood up and removed his cap. After praying, I asked her some questions, because I saw that she has lost her pregnancy. She then told me that for 4 consecutive times, she has gotten pregnant, and on a particular day and time a man comes and violates her at night. And a day later she will start bleeding. She said it happened before she came. She has gone to all kinds of spiritual houses to solve the problem. Had all kinds of rituals done o her to no avail. I told her, that she will have to break all those negative spiritual influences and free herself.

People want short cut. We started the process but she will have to complete it.

CHAPTER 4

BREAKING YOKES OF INFERTLITY

4.1. A Personal Story

My family from the father's side, worshipped the sea goddess. I still wonder if they knew it. She is called Liengu. Some families have people, usually women who have gone through the Liengu ritual. When the spirit comes to make it's demands, the person she wants switches mode as I called it. She no longer communicates with human tongues. She starts speaking in a strange tongue. One that can only be interpreted only by a child that is learning to speak. She will be incubated as if it were for a period of nine months. With specific instructions on diets, sleeping habits and so on. Other liengus are the only ones allowed to attend to her. During this period, she will be incubated and lives in isolation. No social activities. And after the period of nine months, she will be taken to the river side; in my place they usually use the beach for this ritual. Back then, it was a touristic event. The Liengu dance. Or the dance of the Liengu.

Different tribes have different names for this Diety. As a young child, I was very curious. My grand dad was a priest and my grand mother a Liengu. (I don't think they knew the implications). All they know is that it is part of the Bakweri culture. Take for example the nude ritual that a pregnant traditional bakweri woman has to do when she carries her first pregnancy. A ritual is done in the forest and then she walks in to the village stark naked. I witnessed it once. That if she doesn't do it, "country fashion" will haunt her unborn child. So a child even before he or she is born has been sold out. Later in life as an adult, when things starts happening, no one remembers that event not to mention connecting their live's challenges to rituals like that. And instead of breaking the covenants, spiritual charlatans starts feeding on them.

In the realm of the spirit, the Liengu dance represent the peak of celebration and final possession of a person by the Sea goddess. In the Bakweri land it is a privilege to be chosen. I was quite young when I discovered that I had a problem. With all the nocturnal visitors I was having, and so many other things. Sometimes I will wake up in another place dressed in strange silk gowns. Made from materials I have never seen in real life. Growing up, they started making demands on me. Because claims were I was royalty in the water kingdom with duties to fulfill. At seventeen, I had a special visit from a creature called Migdal. Claiming he was my husband. He had human form except for the fact that he was a giant. Abnormally tall and huge. I was not to marry a human and worse, I was not to have human kids. My family saw me going through all kinds of spiritual trauma. All kinds of rituals were performed to free me from their demands. Blood sacrifices involving goats, fowls and other things. I eat drank and had all kinds of thing put inside of me.

At that time, I didn't know that I was to take over the mantle from my grandma. This so called husband has followed me all my life. And nearly killed me when I eventually got pregnant after eight years with my son's father. I was never meant to have kids. It was violation according to them, and they had to punish me for it. But they failed. Because I had build a positive spirituality. I had become a follower of The Nazarene. I carried/bore on me, The Mark of the Blood. Jesus had become my shield. I was living under a stronger covenant. To protect my child and me, I was given Angelic guards. Special ones. Two of them followed me everywhere I went. Day and nights they protected us. All because, I dare to defy forces that claimed they owned me and broke evil covenants made in ignorance. Even as a believer, they monitored me from a distance. I on another mission. Sent by the Master of the Universe. They has lost their grip over me. And they were furious. In 2003, my son's father fought for my life. I was depressed, severely depressed. From trauma caused by the authoritarian dictatorial man I was following as a pastor. He too demanded that my son's father and I made a covenant, vowing never to have biological children. And we did sealed with a 40 days of fasting without food.. Praying a prayer like, "Lord, we take this vow today never to have biological children so that we would be available for you to send wherever we are needed whenever we are needed." This satanic vow, done in God's name, re-enforced what was done to me as a child. So I went in and out of depressing throughout the time I was with him. So on this particular night, I came home late from caring for a patient. I was staying in her house. But that night, she was on admission. On my way back home, this being followed me mocking. That I should give up the faith, the One I decided to follow has failed me. That it was time to go home and fulfill my responsibility as a princess. I was to go back to my late father's village without letting anyone in my immediate family know that I was in town. The pressure to go was so strong. He followed me until I got to where I was staying. When I got home, took my bath and prepared to sleep; my son's father tried talking to me, then he started praying in tongues and I started laughing. An eerie laughter even in my own ears. But I couldn't control myself. He kept praying, and I started dancing. It was the Liengu dance. My body was completely taken over. I found myself being carried away by Migdal while, my occupied body lay on the floor performing a strange dance. I saw my son's father praying. At some point he wanted to run away. I saw him hesitate at the door. Then he came back and continued praying. With the last straw of faith in me, I started spraying in my spirit. The face on the body in that room wasn't mine; I was being carried away towards what seems to be a stone altar. But I kept praying in my spirit, fighting. At some point, he threw me on the ground and fled with a calabash. But as he did, the calabash fell and got broken. At this point, I came back to myself. Clothes were thorn, looking haggard and completely worn out. That was the night my grandma died as I later learnt. I broke the Liengu linage in my family by refusing the crown. And nearly lost my life in the process. It was a very fierce battle. I will forver be grateful to my on's father for staying. When all he wanted to do was run. He later explained some details to me. How another woman took over my body. And how the Holy Spirit asked him to stay otherwise, it will be my corpse he will meet when he comes back.

Some years later, I got pregnant also through a big fight. Someday during our talk shows on SPIRITUAL DIMENSIONS which will be starting soon, my son's father will share the story of how that part of the covenant was broken. He was instrumental in many ways in my life even though it was also tough on him. He saw me face all kinds of things. My nights were warfare most of the time. As a missionary, I have by the grace of God, helped many women break free from covenants that were done on their behalf or by themselves in ignorance, mitigating against their ability to procreate. And we're still doing that. With the advent of fertility treatment, women have been able to bypass a lot of things and still had children some extreme cases, through surrogacy. But God took me to a place where I had to fight for the lives of these children at a time when they were most fragile. And in all the instances, covenants had to be broken as God kept revealing things concerning their parents. All of which were confirmed. On two different occasions, I was attacked by the spirits involved, who claimed that I had no business getting involved in their affairs. These will be shared in other write–ups.

I received these insides through revelations after given my life to the Lord at nineteen. 12th January 1992. And it's been a very fierce battle.

I had a lot of spiritual experiences during pregnancy. For close to six months I was confined to a single room. Nursing and fighting for the life of the remaining child in her womb. (One of them died in utero in the early stage of the pregnancy). Against medical advice, I decided to the keep the pregnancy irrespective of the outcome. Doctors tried to convince me to evacuate. Since carrying a life and dead fetus to term was packed with high risk. I carried both the life and the dead baby for seven months. And had abdominal pains and vaginal discharges from the day one of the babies died in utero till they were born. One alive, the other dead. No one touched my preterm baby for the first three months of his life including his father and my mother. I had to re-enforce his spiritual hedge.

This was the price I paid for daring to break the unhealthy covenants made on my behalf even before I was born, and the one I made in a spiritually unhealthy relationship with a man who claimed to be a servant of God. Unfortunately, he is till deceiving many till date.

Spiritual healing included repentance for following and obeying a man instead of God, it involved forgiveness of self and others and deliberately breaking vows made. Then daily declarations of God's will for my life as it is written in the Bible; speaking healing scripture life; nullifying negative words spoken to me and against me.

Today, my son is a big boy and I am still involved in the greatest rescue missions of all time. **THE DIVINE RESCUE!**

We will be systematically handling the breaking of yokes, covenants and destruction of satanic altars in the prayer section.

There are two stories I will like to share here. The first one is that of a woman who had a dream after she got pregnant. She said some men dressed in strange robes entered their house one night looking for her husband. They said they have come to kill him for refusing to pay them what he owed them. The woman pleaded with them in the dream. But they insisted they must kill him. She then told them that she was pregnant and asked them to take her unborn child instead. The next day, she had a miscarriage. And have not been able to conceive ever since. Maybe she thought that would be the only child they would take. But every time she gets pregnant, she loses the baby. Satan, the Bible says is a lie from the beginning. He can never tell you the whole story.

The second story is that of a young a friend of mine. I had a dream in which I met her kissing another woman. I rebuked her and woe up. When I prayed for her, the Lord simple asked me to tell her the dream that she will understand. And I did. When I told her, she told me she had lost eight pregnancies during the course of her marriage because a particular woman violates her at three months of every pregnancy until she loses the pregnancy. Until a day when she cried out to God and fought this being with the Word of God. She then told me that she was pregnant and the being has been threatening. That's when I prayed with her throughout the pregnancy until she had her baby. That was her third child. Alleluia! There is victory in Jesus Name! We will handle this in the prayer section.

CHAPTER 5

TAKING YOUR SEED

5.1. My Testimony

After eight years of marriage, I got a job in one hospital Ajayi Medical Centre in Ikorodu Lagos Nigeria. Within a few months of work, I started having patients showing their gratitude to me through prayers. They always prayed blessed me with my own children. And insists in their prayers that God should bless me with twins. It was the first time that I ever wished I had a child. I had never really had that longing. I had already made arrangements to adopt a child. A friend who was pregnant had agreed to give me her last baby. She had five kids already.

But a few months into the job, I started falling sick on and off. Got treated on and of for malaria. At some point I dared to do a pregnancy test with urine and home. It came out positive. Since I wasn't expecting to get pregnant, I went to the hospital to do a blood test. It came and positive. Our gynecologist decided to do a scan based on the number of weeks I had been sick. Results, I saw two babies inside of me! At 36 years, no medication apart from a supplement I was taking for fibroids. Can't even remember the name. I got pregnant just like that. It was too good to be true. But it was also the beginning of trouble for me.

I had two covenants working against me. The Liengu covenant and one I took as a believer. The man, who was playing the role of my mentor, had gotten my son's father and I take a vow to never have biological children. We were supposed to make ourselves available to God 24/7 to be sent anywhere anytime for the preaching of the gospel. It is a long story and this is not the place to share that. What I want to share her are the spiritual encounters I had during the pregnancy.

I had a series of physical attacks with invisible hands pulling me from the bed. Right infront of Mandi. I will beg him to pray and he will simple look at me with glassy eyes and tell me that he is praying inside of him. Sometimes I will simply feel hands on my stomach squeezing and someone asking me how I managed to get pregnant. Twice I dreamed of my dead relatives coming and trying squeeze the child out of me. I was at war to protect y unborn babies.

5.2. Angelic Guides

When the stakes gets high, God brings in the Angelic factor. After some time, I started noticing two beings walking beside me. I could only see their white wings. When I start feeling the pain, they would touch me slightly with their wings. Sometimes it felt like I was hidden inside of them. I felt safe. One day, I can't remember if I was awake or asleep. But I found myself on a strange journey. I couldn't the person beside me. but he said he was one of the babies in my womb. He took me to a big hall. It was like a very long room. Endless it seems. With countless number of doors on both side. he called the place treasure house. He said everyone one earth has their own room. And the room contains everything they will need for their lives on earth. Each door had a name. told me that before The Father sends anyone on earth, he had prepared all their resources. Then all of a sudden, he asked it would like to see mine. I told him sure. Some doors were wide open, others partially opened, some sealed, and so on. As we were moving, he said those closed doors are belonged to some who have not been sent to earth yet while others belonged to those we call poor. They lack the faith to access their resources, there are details I wouldn't go into here. He finally stopped in-front of a door that was partially open. And told me that was my own treasure room. He explained why it was partially open. I could peep in and see what seems like a room filled with indescribable wealth. I will stop here. He then took me to another door. And told me that was his. And I suddenly found myself on my bed.

5.3. I Finished My Mission

Another day, I had another visit. This time, it was the other twin. He told me it was time for him to go back to The Father. That he has finished his mission. He said The Father asked him to accompany his brother to earth because the battle over his birth was too heavy. But that he had to be born. He went ahead and explained his brother's mission and told me some other things. He said he had a favor to ask me. That I should not tell his twin brother that he died. Because he didn't die. He simply finished his own mission. How can he be dead when I saw them moving in my womb some days back? My gynaecologist always joking told me that my babies are moving at a time when fetuses shouldn't be active. They were surrounded by five huge fibroids. They were acting like they were pushing the fibroids away from themselves. He will say, your babies are acting as if they were fighting demons. I will stop here on this one.

In yet another encounter, my angel guide came and simply told me that he want to take me to a place. We walked for what seemed to have been ages in the heart of a thick forest until we found ourselves in front of a gate. A big gate. Most times we simply float in the air. Sometimes we walked. On this particular day, it was as if the journey had no end. But finally here we were, in front of this big gate. He then asked me to go in. I looked at him and wondered why he wasn't coming with me. he told me, his own part of the journey ended there. That he cannot go in with me but that he would be waiting for me. For one last time, I looked at this giant angel and the faced what seems like an inevitable journey I must embark on. I pushed and entered the compound. Trees everywhere, but there was a path. So I followed the path. But there was no end in view. Only trees and a hushed silence as if the trees were alive. Could see, feel and even talk. As if they were watching my every move. But I was not afraid. Because somehow, I knew I couldn't escape they journey. After what seems like an endless journey, I sudden saw ahead of me a very high fence. And attached to the fence were rails. From the floor till close to the top of the fence. The whole stretch of that fence had these rails. They were like endless. As I got closer, I noticed that behind them were babies! All lying on each other. If you have ever witness a maggot nest, you will begin to grasp what I am describing. Like we have hundreds of thousands of babies lying on each other moving like a nest of maggot, countless number of them. then the Angel started speaking. He told me to take mine and leave. That once I carry mine, I should run without turning. Again, I pushed open one of the inner gates that hosted the babies and carried one of them. somehow, I knew I was pregnant with twins, yet all I took was one baby. Immediately I touched the baby, the trees became creatures. Some half goat half human with long tails, creatures and beast walking on two legs, following me yet unable to touch me. they were making strange sounds. I ran for dear life. holding my baby close. The Angel kept saying run until you are out of the gate. These ones are territorial. They can't go beyond that gate. Keep running. Can't tell why they couldn't touch me. I finally got to the gate, pushed and ran out. They came and stopped at the gate. Stretching to touch me but couldn't. within moments, once again it was just a forest.

So I asked the angel what that meant, he told me that these are children of some of those women we call barren on earth. He told me that there is no woman born barren. That they just didn't know how to take their babies. For many reasons, some of which I have mentioned before, their fruit became caged in places like this. But that these demons cannot stop anyone who get to the point of entering to collect their babies. He also told me that each woman has a different thing to do to break forth and take their babies just as each one's babies got there in the first place for a different reason. He said some women spend their time praying, fasting, when all they need was simple acts of kindness. Not just generosity. But kindness. He said a lot of things while bring me back home.   Finally I woke up. And instinctively touched my stomach. I knew immediately that I wouldn't be giving birth to twins. I kept quite. Went to do a repeat scan, and a huge fibroid was sitting on the head of the second twin. The other one was quite.

I spent over 80% of the 7 months/28weeks of the pregnancy in the hospital. A was bleeding throughout. First reddish, then brownish stuff with particles were coming out of me. The doctors tried to convince me to evacuate but I refused. I signed against medical advice. I went through the pain. They planned a Caeserian section at week 28. A week to the day, the Lord asked me to tell OA to bring the babies stuff. That I will not be doing a CS. He was mad, rebuked me for being stubborn. Why I'm I insisting on natural delivery with a dead and a life baby inside of me. By this time, the kind of pain I have been through meant that I couldn't talk much. So I begged OA to simply bring the things and we will allow the doctors do what they have to do. I worked in the hospital in my pain. Attended to patients during night shift. Helped and comforted anyone who needed help or comfort. I was in the private ward in Ajayi medical centre Ikorodu. I will never forget doctor Ajayi and what he did for me.

On the seventh day after that encounter with the lord, the labour pain increased. Doctor Oni said he will section me if i do not deliver within 24 hours. I was a high risk patient. For hours i stayed on 4cm. The labour monitor said I was ready. But I was just 4cm; eventually they left me. After a while, I became pressed with urine. Went in and emptied my bladder, when I came back into the room, I felt the pressure of something coming out of me. One of the nurses was with me the doctor had just left. So I lowered myself to the floor thinking that the baby was about dropping off me. Once on the floor, because the bed was too high for me, a huge balloon-like stuff came out of me. By this time, the doctor had been called. He spoke in Yoruba. And it was a question he asked. Like what is this? As they tried lifting me, the balloon thing busted spilling an odourless brownish fluid all over the place. My own sac came all the way and spill off the fluid filled with the particles from the skin of the dead baby. All the while, my Angelic guides stood by my. Their brightness was unbelievable. Whenever they allow me to see a glimpse of the wings, it took me days to recover. It felt like I have been staring at the sun. So even in this dark hour of pain, they stood by me one on the both side of the labor couch. Somehow, at some point, I could look at them without blinking.OA stood beside one of them by the wall side of the labor room. But he wasn't even aware of their presence. Their presence helped me deal with the pain. I was simply groaning silently. No progress. They were getting set to take me to the theatre. The doctor has just checked me for what he said would be the last time. He removed one of his gloves, while he was removing the second one. I told him that the baby was coming out. He patiently but firmly made me understood that he has just checked and I was till 4cm. He was facing the sink with his back to me. I kept repeating very slowing because I was too weak to scream, doc the baby is coming out. So he turned, and indeed my baby nearly fell on the floor. He was a very tiny little bundle. So tiny that we could see traces of his ribs. A few minutes later, the dead brother came out, parts of his skin peeled off.

I will save the rest of the story for another time. Here was I 36years old holding the baby I risked my life for. Because I believed God's promises and the visions and dreams, the Angels, the conversations, the warfare, I knew that child had to be born. He is 11 going to 12. He has been one of the reasons I could go on when darkness closed in on me. I would remember everything (some of which I cannot afford to put into writing) God took me through, and know I had to keep moving!

I have ever since ministered to more than 20 women. Most of whom hardly knows my name. God takes me to specific hospitals for specific reasons and for specific seasons. He shows me the people I must minister to. And he tells me when to leave. Some of my colleagues knows what I was doing and would direct people to me. for special prayers.

There are deeper issues involved in this warfare humanity is involved in. Each person should therefore face their battle with tenacity, boldness, courage. And most especially from a stand point of victory. Not from the victim's position.

5.4. The Stakes and the Battle Over Human Procreation

At some point in time along the fertility journey, every woman dealing with infertility has to stop seeing themselves the way the world sees them; as failures, incomplete or useless. As women, our usefulness does not lie solely in our ability to conceive. It lies in our ability to nurture, to create, to cultivate, to build, to strengthen. We are very powerful beings.

We are first and foremost helpers. Unlike the global misconception of who a helper is, the true meaning of a helper is one who supports. And that is why Satan had to first of all neutralize the woman in order to gain access into our race.Destroy humanity by weakening man's Helper. If Satan came through Adam, the woman would have fought back! So she had to be used.

And the distortion that came after the fall changed the role of the woman and relegated her to the minor, lesser, weaker creature only meant to be used s tools. The description of Paul about the woman being a weaker vessel had nothing to do with her inner capacities. It had to do with her physique.

To the use of a woman falls under the category of objects of;
- Pleasure
- Advertisement
- Marketing
- Procreation
- Maids

And a woman will feel hopelessly useless if she fails in any of these with the biggest failure of all being the inability to conceive. Even those who chooses perversion as a way of life, like homosexual or all the perverse sexualities we now have in our era, still want to play the motherhood role. Something is missing if they fail there it seems.

Womanhood and Feminity is equivalent to virtue meaning Power!

- The power to give and receive pleasure
- The power to conceive and nurture a pregnancy
- The power to bring forth another and to nurture a child to adulthood
- The power to mould destines
- The power to build homes and nations and influence kingdoms.

Therefore, there is a need to create a distinction between human traditions including religious ones and the Word of God. According to the word of God,

Your qualifications as God's vice –Reagent does not depend on whether or not you can conceive; as awesome as that experience is. Your qualification depends on God's view of who you are.

- Qualified by God's original design (Gen 2:18; Gen 1:26-28)
- Qualified by redemption in Christ (Gal 3:28)
- Qualified by Jesus example
- Qualified by the examples of the early church(
- Qualified by the word (John 1:12-13, Rom 8:17; 1 Peter 3:7)
- Qualified by opportunity(Lk 8, Lk 10; Isaiah 8:3; Judges 4:5; 2kings 22:14)
- Mercy said No (John 3:16)

All these scripture brought out women who played key role in God's Divine Agenda for Mankind irrespective of Gender or procreation. Who knows Prophetess Deborah's children? But we knew her husband Lapidoth.

5.5. Different Roles the Same Mission

Functionally, the man was created the head while the woman was to be a "helper fit or suitable" to the man. It is a matter of roles.

The word helper have been interpreted in different ways through the ages. From a woman being weaker inferior or simply glorified animal in some cultures. However, the Hebrew word helper (ezer) occurred twenty one times in the Old Testament and seventy one times in the New Testament usually describing the Role of the Holy Spirit as our Helper.

It was only used five times to speak of people helping people. The other sixteen times, it was used as a reference for God as a helper to his people. *It was a superior, more capable being helping a lesser person.* It is also used to describe someone bringing fulfillment, satisfaction to another. She was endowed with extra-ordinary abilities so that she could fulfill her role as "helper suitable" for her man.

But she was to work under control. She was to submit to Adam as head. It is not an easy task to be called to lead a being with such awesome powers. But Adam in addition to all he had to do was to play the role of Eve's protector and guardian. Help her use her gifts for the good of all creation and the glory of God. Eve was to bring in all she had to help Adam succeed to the glory of God. God's interest, Kingdom interest was all that really mattered. But in the process, they were to enjoy one another's presence and person. They were to share in the wonder of creation through the **"Birth Process"** and the pleasure and power of communion through sexual intercourse. It was a wonderful arrangement. Everyone was happy, no inferiority or superiority complexes, no gender confusion, everyone knew their role. Now God was happy and enjoyed His times of fellowship with both Adam and Eve. **And God saw everything that he had made, and, behold, it was very good. And the evening and the morning were the sixth day. (Genesis 1:31).**

But there was Darkness to reckon with. The highest Angel in rank was around. Burning with jealousy for these lovers of God. No he will not fold his arm and watch God lavish His love on creatures he considers inferior to himself. And so he set into motion his second battle for conquest. He failed in Heaven, therefore he was bent on succeeding in his second "Coup D'état". Again he failed. Because only the Omnipotent Omniscient and Omnipresent God, Elohim knew that, injected into creation was the Gene of Redemption! Mankind on like fallen Angel could be redeemed. (Gen 3:15). Thounands of years later after many failed attempts to stop the birth of the Messaiah, Jesus Christ came. Born of a virgin through the Divine Conception. And on the Cross of Calvary, defeated the Devil once and for all. On the cross He Declared, It I Finished! Death has been vanquished! Now Satan's man agenda is to populate hell, his eternal place of doom. Having lived in heaven and coveted the eternal throne of the universe, he knows the true meaning of hell. Beyond the flames: The everlasting separation from God. He delights in spiting God by using mankind, the very object of God's love to fight God.

The battle line ranges is over who rule on earth, Satan and his Dark Horde through the rule of Lawlessness, or Man as God's Vice Regents imposing the rule of Righteousness on Earth. His Target, control the very essence of God's mandate to us. But more so, who rule in the hearts of men. Mammon (Satan) or God.

1. **(Gen 1:26):** And God said, Let us make man in our image, after our likeness: and let them have dominion over the fish of the sea, and over the fowl of the air, and over the cattle, and over all the earth, and over every creeping thing that creeps on the earth.

2. **(Gen 1:27):** So God created man in his own image, in the image of God created he him; male and female created he them.

3. **(Gen 1:28):** And God blessed them, and God said to them, Be fruitful, and multiply, and replenish the earth, and subdue it: and have dominion over the fish of the sea,

and over the fowl of the air, and over every living thing that moves on the earth.

The key words here are;
- Dominion
- Subdue
- Rule
- Replenish
- Multiply
- Fruitfulness
- Blessed
- Likeness
- Image

So irrespective of what anyone tells you as a woman, you have the God-seed in you. Approach your challenge with fertility as part of your battle. And woe betides you if you entered the battle with the mindset of a failure.

There is war on earth over who rules. The devil wants to decide who rules, how and with whom we have sex, who and why we marry, how we procreate, how, when and whether or not we should multiply. He is creating the chaos, so that he can bring his own kind of solutions. As women, we must begin to view ourselves and our mission as bigger than just marriage and child birth. If we miss out on the Whys, we will also miss out on the Hows, the Wheres and the Whens. We must therefore rediscover our true mission as Women and Re-awaken the Helper Spirit in us. And push back the Devil from our individual space, our community, our nations and our world. We can do it. We must do it.

If you must conceive, approach your journey from the position of victory. Motherhood is your Divine Heritage. The Devil is only a Thief, a murderer and destroyer. You can reclaim your Fertility as well as all your other God-Given Capacity as a "Helper Spirit. So much is at stake.

CHAPTER 6

GODS PROMISES TO ANSWER PRAYERS

Mathew 21:22: "*If you believe, you will receive whatever you ask for in prayer.*" *So I say to you: Ask and it will be given to you; seek and you will find; knock and the door will be opened to you. For everyone who asks receives; the one who seeks finds; and to the one who knocks, the door will be opened. Which of you fathers, if your son asks for a fish, will give him a snake instead? Or if he asks for an egg, will give him a scorpion? If you then, though you are evil, know how to give good gifts to your children, how much more will your Father in heaven give the Holy Spirit to those who ask him! If you declare with your mouth, "Jesus is Lord," and believe in your heart that God raised him from the dead, you will be saved. 10 For it is with your heart that you believe and are justified, and it is with your mouth that you profess your faith and are saved.*

Proverbs 3:5-6: *Trust in the Lord with all your heart and lean not on your own understanding; in all your ways submit to him, and he will make your paths straight.*

John 8:12: *I am the light of the world. Whoever follows me will never walk in darkness, but will have the light of life.*

Luke 11:9-13: *So I say to you: Ask and it will be given to you; seek and you will find; knock and the door will be opened to you. For everyone who asks receives; the one who seeks finds; and to the one who knocks, the door will be opened. Which of you fathers, if your son asks for a fish, will give him a snake instead? Or if he asks for an egg, will give him a scorpion? If you then, though you are evil, know how to give good gifts to your children, how much more will your Father in heaven give the Holy Spirit to those who ask him!*

Romans 10:9-10: *If you declare with your mouth, "Jesus is Lord," and believe in your heart that God raised him from the dead, you will be saved. 10 For it is with your heart that you believe and are justified, and it is with your mouth that you profess your faith and are saved.*

6.1. Scriptural Back Up On Infertility

Psalms 113:9 - He maketh the barren woman to keep house, [and to be] a joyful mother of children. Praise ye the LORD.

Mark 11:24 - Therefore I say unto you, What things soever ye desire, when ye pray, believe that ye receive [them], and ye shall have [them].

John 16:33 - These things I have spoken unto you, that in me ye might have peace. In the world ye shall have tribulation: but be of good cheer; I have overcome the world.

1 Samuel 1:1-28 - Now there was a certain man of Ramathaimzophim, of mount Ephraim, and his name [was] Elkanah, the son of Jeroham, the son of Elihu, the son of Tohu, the son of Zuph, an Ephrathite:

Romans 5:3-5 - And not only [so], but we glory in tribulations also: knowing that tribulation worketh patience;

Romans 12:12 - Rejoicing in hope; patient in tribulation; continuing instant in prayer;

Hebrews 11:11 - Through faith also Sara herself received strength to conceive seed, and was delivered of a child when she was past age, because she judged him faithful who had promised.

Psalms 139:13 - For thou hast possessed my reins: thou hast covered me in my mother's womb.

Psalms 127:3 - Lo, children [are] an heritage of the LORD: [and] the fruit of the womb [is his] reward.

Genesis 25:21 - And Isaac entreated the LORD for his wife, because she [was] barren: and the LORD was entreated of him, and Rebekah his wife conceived.

Psalms 147:3 - He healeth the broken in heart, and bindeth up their wounds.

Luke 1:36-37 - And, behold, thy cousin Elisabeth, she hath also conceived a son in her old age: and this is the sixth month with her, who was called barren. (Read

Psalms 128:3 - Thy wife [shall be] as a fruitful vine by the sides of thine house: thy children like olive plants round about thy table.

Deuteronomy 7:14 - Thou shalt be blessed above all people: there shall not be male or female barren among you, or among your cattle.

Isaiah 54:1-17 - Sing, O barren, thou [that] didst not bear; break forth into singing, and cry aloud, thou [that] didst not travail with child: for more [are] the children of the desolate than the children of the married wife, saith the LORD. (Read More...)

Philippians 4:13 - I can do all things through Christ which strengtheneth me.

1 Samuel 2:21 - And the LORD visited Hannah, so that

she conceived, and bare three sons and two daughters. And the child Samuel grew before the LORD.

Genesis 1:28 - And God blessed them, and God said unto them, Be fruitful, and multiply, and replenish the earth, and subdue it: and have dominion over the fish of the sea, and over the fowl of the air, and over every living thing that moveth upon the earth.

Exodus 23:26 - There shall nothing cast their young, nor be barren, in thy land: the number of thy days I will fulfil.

Genesis 25:21 And Isaac prayed to the Lord for his wife, because she was barren. And the Lord granted his prayer, and Rebekah his wife conceived.

6.2. Repentance

- **Acts 3:19:** Repent, then, and turn to God, so that your sins may be wiped out, that times of refreshing may come from the Lord.
- **Proverbs 28:13:**Whoever conceals their sins does not prosper, but the one who confesses and renounces them finds mercy.

Repentance takes away from the devil his power to inject doubts in your hearts during prayer. Apart from receiving access to the Father through Christ, the Bible calls him the accuser. If he has nothing to hold on to, his accusations will bounce. You can approach the throne of Grace and Mercy with faith, boldness and courage as well as humility.By the New and living way; The Blood of Jesus Christ we can have access to God.

So search your heart, deal with guilt. When Adam and Eve sinned, they hid from God's presence. You cannot honestly enter God's presence with clouds of sin. So repent and ask for forgiveness for known and unknown sins.

You can't afford to enter the battle field, breaking and demolishing strongholds that have been working against your fertility with uncleanness. If you do that, you will re-enforce their grip on you. And of course block your own break through.

6.3. Praying Through Fertility

Repentance From all kinds of sins; Sexual sins, bitterness, hatred, perversion, masturbation, pornography, adultery, idolatory, witchcraft, jealousy, envy (how can they have children while I am still struggling), covetousness (you are coveting another's spouse because you think they are fertile and yours is not), emotional unfaithfulness. You know those secret sins, dig them out! Repent and throw them off. Receive forgiveness, cleansing, healing and restoration. You've been carrying the baggage of in for too long. Drop it off! It is time to enter a new era in your life. And you cannot afford to enter with unnecessary baggage.

6.4. Exhortation

The enemy can go to any length using any tool to attack us in many ways. Our physical health, our souls, even our spirit man. Remember do not concentrate on any human being. As you break down strongholds God will handle the rest. (no names, no sending of fire to destroy any one). He can attack any internal or external organ in our bodies including our reproductive organ with deformity, diseases and mal-functioning. God is able to deliver you and turn your situation around irrespective of the medical terminology used. I have many personal testimonies of God's divine healing. And I know many people who have also received medical miracles from different kinds of diseases and disorder including infertility.

Yours will not be different In Jesus Name. Amen!

6.5. General Thanksgiving

1. Thank God for life.

2. Thank God for your husband/wife.

3. Thank God for your wards.

4. Thank God for all His goodness in your life.

5. Thank him for His presence in your life.

6. Give Him praise for His love and mercies towards you.

7. Give Him glory for His everlasting covenant made with the blood of His only begotten son Jesus Christ.

8. Worship Him in your own words.

9. Pour your heart out to Him in praise. For He inhabits our praise

10. Pray in known and unknown tongues.

6.6. Speaking God's Words In Your Specific Situation

1 Peter 2:24: He personally carried our sins in his body on the cross so that we can be dead to sin and live for what is right. But his wounds you are healed.

Jeremiah 30:17: "I will give you back your health and heal your wounds," says the Lord.

Isaiah 53:5 : But he was pierced for our rebellion, crushed for our sins. He was beaten so we could be whole. He was whipped so we could be healed.

Psalm 41:3: The Lord nurses them when they are sick and restores them to health.

Psalm 103:2-3: Let all that I am praise the Lord; may I never forget the good things he does for me. He forgives all my sins and heals all my diseases.

Psalm 6:2: Have compassion on me, Lord, for I am weak. Heal me, Lord, for my bones are in agony.

6.7. Breaking Down and Rebuilding

- Annul every decree that contradicts God's plan for you to have your own baby in the Name of Jesus Christ.
- Through Christ we have been redeemed by a New Covenant. The Covenant sealed with the Blood of Jesus Christ. Therefore in the Name of Jesus Christ, cancel every other covenant irrespective of who made it and how it was made that speaks contrary to God's Divine plan for your life concerning fertility.
- If ever altars were built with you and you fruits mentioned, in the Name of Jesus Shatter the altar and cancel it's effect where ever it is. Pray in your own words, pouring your heart out to God. Lay hold of His plans for your life. Plans for good and not evil. To bring you to an expected end.
- Strongholds working against you and yours, in the Name of Jesus Christ we nullify their effect, we break their grip, we disconnect you from them in Jesus Name. Pray in the spirit. Victory is yours in Jesus Name.
- In the name of Jesus Christ free yourselves as a couple from spirits of infirmity, deformity and infertility, bareness.
- Pray for the restoration of ovaries, uterus, Fallopian tubes, cervix and all their functions to return to normal.
- Pray for your spouse.
- Begin to decree good things.
- Decree that all your reproductive organs were created by a God who has spares. He has the power to restore structure and function. Call Him to restore all your organs. The functioning of all systems related to reproduction including hormones.
- Lay hands on your abdomen below your navel and speak wellness, wholesomeness to your reproductive organs.

- Command your womb to carry and nurture your baby. In the Name of Jesus Christ!
- Get your husband to seal these prayers. Let it be a couple's fight. Let him play the priest role in his home. And speak with authority. Satan understands hierarchy. If your husband stand his ground as head, Satan will give way. He will shift. It is the law of Hierarchy. Alleluia! Alleluia! Alleluia!
- **The Bible says, Isaac prayed for his barren wife and she conceived. Hierarchy.**

6.8. Praying Through Fertility: Positive

Confessions and Decrees

PRAYER 1.

Then I said, "Please, O LORD God of heaven, great and awesome God, who keeps his loving covenant with those who love him and obey his commandments. **Neh 1:5**

Father, as Your children, we come before You and remind You that we have been redeemed from the curse of the law, we have been delivered from sin and all it's consequences and You have promised us all the blessings of Abraham. We are in a covenant with You, and we expect You to fulfill the conditions of that covenant.

PRAYER 2.

I praise you, for I am fearfully and wonderfully made. Wonderful are your works; my soul knows it very well. **Psalm 139:14**

Father, we desire to have a baby, and since Your Word says that children are a gift from You, we expect a normal, healthy baby to be sent to us.

As a husband, for my wife (her name) has been redeemed from the curse, we expect her to carry that child full term. Your Word says You will bless the fruit of my womb, and Your Word says I will lose none of my young by miscarriage or be barren, and that You will keep me safe through childbearing. Since I am no longer under the curse, I will be able to have this child the way You originally planned Eve to have children free from pain and suffering, and pangs and spasms of distress. So, as a couple we expect this child to be brought into the world quickly and with no pain. As a husband I believe she will feel the contractions but not pain. We believe, according to Your Word, that she will have a beautiful pregnancy with no suffering during it.

Thank You, Father, for hearing and answering our prayers and for faithfully watching over Your Word to perform it. We know You have given Your angels charge over us to accompany and defend and preserve us in all our ways. Amen.

PRAYER 3

Lo, **children are a heritage of the Lord**: and the fruit of the womb **is** his reward. **Psalm 127:3, KJV**

Father, we thank You that children are the heritage of the Lord, fertility prayer and the fruit of the womb is His reward. Children are Your idea, Father; You thought up children, and family, and home You instituted the family in the Garden of Eden. You ordered children; You commanded them when You said to Adam and Eve, "Be fruitful and multiply." You said that the barren womb is never satisfied. Lord, the Word declares that I am wonderfully and fearfully made by You; therefore, I'm perfect and able to conceive and have children. Please give me the opportunity to carry out this blessing and use this magically gift to create my own family. In the Name of Jesus Christ.

PRAYER 4

Praise the Lord for He is great, mighty, and gives life. May He remember me as He did Sarah, planting seed in my womb, bearing fruit, as the most bountiful tree in the orchard. (And the LORD visited Sarah as He had said, and the LORD did for Sarah as He had spoken.)

Lord on high, Lord so close, make me fertile. Create a new soul and I will raise it up in Your name. Hallelujah!

PRAYER 5

I praise you, for I am fearfully and wonderfully made. Wonderful are your works; my soul knows it very well. Psalm 139:14

Fertility is within my reach. I close my eyes and see conception. Carefully, I will nurture God's greatest creation, a new life. I am ready, willing, and able to bear a child. The Lord is with me. I will walk with confidence along the path where mothers before me have walked. The time for getting pregnant is here. My prayers will be answered. It is God's will.

Thank you, Lord, for all the blessings in my life. Help me to remember them as I face the challenges of infertility. I pray that I can surrender myself into your hands. Let me accept the reality of this situation and have the wisdom and courage to take action where I can the way You want me to. Strengthen my body, mind and spirit to endure the trials of infertility. Keep me ever mindful of the needs of others and grant us your peace in Jesus Name. Amen.

PRAYER 6

13 For you created my inmost being; you knit me together in my mother's womb. **14** I praise you because I am fearfully and wonderfully made; your works are wonderful, I know that full well. **15** My frame was not hidden from you when I was made in the secret place, when I was woven together in the depths of the earth. **16** Your eyes saw my unformed body; all the days ordained for me were written in your book before one of them came to be. **Psalm 139:13-16**

Loving Father I am fearfully and wonderfully made and I thank and praise You that You knew me before I was conceived in my mother's womb. You formed and knitted me together and breathed life into me.

PRAYER 7

Now this is the confidence that we have in Him, that if we ask anything according to His will, He hears us. **I John 5:14**

Father You told Your children to be fruitful and multiply and I long to carry my own child in my womb and hold my own precious babe in my arms, but I have not yet conceived and this grieves and hurts me deeply. I come to You as You daughter asking for You intervention.

PRAYER 8

I will be your God throughout your lifetime – until your hair is white with age. I made you, and I will care for you. I will carry you along and save you. **Isaiah 46:4**

Loving Lord I know that You have scheduled every day of my life and I pray that in Your goodness and grace You will enable me to conceive and bring into the world a little one that I may give back to You – just as Hannah gave her Samuel back into Your care. Look down on me in love and compassion and breathe into my barren womb, the breath of life, which was breathed into man at creation and fill me to the fullness of Your joy so that I may bring forth a little baby. I ask this in Jesus name, Amen

PRAYER 9

So do not fear, for I am with you; do not be dismayed, for I am your God. I will strengthen you and help you; I will uphold you with my righteous right hand. **Isaiah 41:10**

Dear Lord, the pain of infertility is so deep. All of our lives, we dream of being mothers, of raising children with loving hearts to do your will on this earth. Month after month when that dream does not come true, it so painful, Lord. We feel like our dreams die each month with empty arms. Please guide us to trust in your plan for us. We desperately need you in our lives. Thank you for all the blessings we do have, knowing through you all things are possible.

PRAYER 10

Dear Lord Jesus, as we walk towards starting a family bless me I pray, with a healthy pregnancy and give us both the wisdom to be good, and wise parents.

May Your will be done in our lives and help us to fulfill our purpose in life by becoming a little family rather than just a couple... O Lord hear my prayer I pray, Amen.

PRAYER 11

Dear Lord I know that children are a heritage and a gift from You.

THANK YOU Lord I know that You are a God that answers prayers and we pray in Jesus name.

PREPARATIONS
- Start thanking god for answered prayers.
- Come up with the names of your kids.
- Start reading books on parenthood.
- Prepare! Prepare! Prepare! Prepare!

Glory be to God!

Watch out for book two.
Praying through the IVF journey (knowing what you want).

INDEX/DEFINITIONS

1. **Abortion:** operation to terminate pregnancy; an operation or other intervention to terminate pregnancy by removing the embryo or fetus from the womb.
2. **Abstinence:** self-denial; restraint from indulging in a desire for something, e.g. alcohol or sexual relations.
3. **Addiction:** A strong and harmful need to regularly have something (such as a drug) or do something (such as gamble) e.g. he has a drug *addiction*.
4. **Adultery:** extramarital sex; voluntary sexual relations between a married person and somebody other than his or her spouse.
5. **Afflictions:** Distress; a condition of great physical or mental distress; cause of distress.
6. **Altar:** Structure on which offerings are made to a deity.
7. **ART:**   Assisted Reproductive Therapies.
8. **Barren:** *of a woman or female animal* not able to produce children or offspring. A *Barren* Woman.
9. **Bisexual:** Attracted to both sexes; sexually attracted to both men and women, or engaging in both heterosexual and homosexual activities
10.   **Bliss:** Complete happiness; perfect happiness. E.g., it was bliss to have a day at home.
11.   **Conceive:** To think of or create (something) in the mind. *Conceive* an idea. A writer who has *conceived* (*imagined*) an entire world of amazing creature.
Or To become pregnant. Or woman who has been unable to *conceive.*

12.   **Conception:** Something conceived in the mind; a result of thoughts, e.g. an idea, invention, or plan.

Biology: the fertilization of an egg by a sperm at the beginning of pregnancy.

Formulation of ideas; the process of arriving at an abstract idea or belief; or the moment at which such an idea starts to take shape or emerge.

13.   **Creator:** A person who makes something new: the *creator* of the popular television show or, the web site's *creators. OR **creator** GOD "all men are endowed by their *creator* with certain unalienable right. *U.S. declaration of independence* (1776)

14.   **Deception:** Practice of misleading someone; the practice of deliberately making someone believe things that are not true.

Something intended to mislead somebody: an act, trick, or device intended to deceive or mislead somebody.

15.   **Desires:** Wish for something; to want something very strongly.

Find somebody sexually attractive; to wish to have sexual relations with somebody.

16.   **Despicable:** worthy of contempt; fully deserving contempt.

17.   **Deviation:** An action, behavior, or condition that is different from what is usual or expected.

18.   **Diabolic**: extremely evil. A *diabolical (fiendish, devilish)* enemy. *Diabolical* often describes a plot, scheme, etc; that is very clever and that is   intended for an evil purpose.

19.   **Distortion:** Misleading alterations: the describing or reporting of something in ways that inaccurate or misleading.

- Configurations from correct shape; the bending, twisting, stretching, or forcing of something out of its usual or natural shape.

- Misshapen parts; parts of something which have been bent, twisted, stretched, or forced out of its usual or natural shape.

20. **Dominion:** Ruling control; ruling power, authority, or control.

Sphere of influence; somebody's area of influence or control. Land ruled; the land governed by a ruler (sometimes used in the plural form, e.g., the monarch's dominions beyond the sea).

21. **Emancipation:** The act of getting or granting freedom; the act or process of setting someone free, or of freeing somebody from restrictions.

Being freed; the condition or fact of being set free or freed from some restrictions.

22. **Feminism:** The belief that men and women should have equal rights and opportunities. Or; organized activity in support of women's rights and interests

23. **Gender:** An individual's gender; the sex of a person (male or female), or organism, or of a whole category of people or organisms (sometimes preferred while trying to avoid using the word "sex").

24. **Helper:** Someone who helps another person with a job or task. E.g The carpenter measured the wall while one of his *helpers* brought in the tools.

25. **Holistic:** Analyzing a whole system of beliefs; characterized by the view that a

whole system of beliefs must be analyzed rather than simply done in its

individual components.

Considering all factors when treating an illness; taking into account all of a patient's physical, mental, and social conditions in the treatment of illness

26. **Immortal:** Never dying; able to have eternal

life or existence.
Famous; very famous and likely to be remembered for a long time.

27. **Incest:** Sex between close relatives; sexual activity between two people who for moral, genetic or religious reasons are considered too closely related to have such a relationship.

28. **Infertility:** Infertility is usually defined as the inability of a couple to achieve a pregnancy after repeated intercourse without contraception for 1 year.

29. **Sexual Intercourse:** Sex involving penetration; an act carried out for reproduction or pleasure involving penetration, especially one in which a man inserts his erect penis inside a woman's vagina.

30. **IVF:** In Vitro Fertilization

31. **Lust:** Sexual desire; the strong physical desire to have sex with someone,
usually without associated feelings of love or affection.
Eagerness; great eagerness or enthusiasm for something; a lust for power.

32. **Menopause:** the time in a woman's life when blood stops flowing from her body each month. The time when a woman stops menstruating.

33. **Nudity:** Being unclothed; the state of having no clothes on. Bareness or plainness, with no covering or decoration.

34. **Nullify:** To make (something) legally null. Or To cause (something) to lose its value or to have no effect.

35. **Nurture:** To help (something or someone) to grow, develop, or succeed. E.g Teachers should *nurture* their students' creativity.
  • To take care of (someone or something that is

growing or developing) by providing food, protection, a place to live, etc. The study looks at the ways parents *nurture* their children.

- To hold (something, such as an idea or a strong feeling) in your mind for a long time. She *nurtured* a secret ambition to be a singer.

36.   Occultism: Belief in supernatural forces; the belief in and study of magic, witchcraft, or supernatural phenomena.

37.   Obsession: A state in which someone thinks about someone or something constantly or frequently especially in a way that is not normal. E.g she has an *obsession* about cleanliness.

- Someone or something that a person thinks about constantly or frequently money has become an *obsession* for him.

38.   Perversion: Unusual sexual practice; a sexual practice considered unusual or unacceptable.

- Turning of good into bad; the changing of something good, true, or correct into something bad or wrong, or a situation in which the change has occurred.

39.   Pleasure: Happiness or satisfaction; a feeling of happiness, delight, or satisfaction.

- Sensual gratification; gratification of the senses, especially sexual gratification.
- Recreation; recreation, relaxation, or amusement, especially as distinct from work or everyday routine.
- Something satisfying; a source of happiness, joy, or satisfaction.
- Somebody's desire; someone's desire or preference.

40.   Procreation: Have offspring; to produce offspring by reproduction. Create something; to create or produce something.

41.   Promiscuity: Undiscriminating sexual behavior; behavior characterized by casual and indiscriminate sexual intercourse, often with many people.

42.   Propagate: Reproduce organism; to reproduce a plant or animal or cause one to reproduce.

- Spread something widely; to spread an idea or custom to many people.

43.   Rape: Forcing someone into sex; the crime of using force on a person for sexual intercourse.

- Instance of rape; an instance of the crime of rape.
- Violent destructive treatment; the violent, destructive, or abusive treatment of something.

44.   Replenish: To make something full again, or to bring it back to it's previous level by replacing what has been used.

45.   Robots: Programmable machine for performing tasks; a mechanical device that can be programmed to carry out instructions and perform complicated tasks usually done by people.

- Imaginary machine; a machine that resembles a human in appearance and can function like a human, especially in science fiction.
- Person behaving like a machine; somebody who works or behaves mechanically and emotionlessly.

46.   Sexism: Sex discrimination; discrimination against women or men because of their sex.

- Sexual stereotyping; the tendency to treat people as cultural stereotypes of their sexes.

47.   Sexuality: State of being sexual; the state of being sexual. Involvement in sexual activities: involvement or interest in sexual activities. Sexual appeal; sexual appeal or potency.

48.   Sovereignty: The full right and power of a governing body over itself, without any interference from outside sources or bodies.

- In spiritual terms, God's Sovereignty or Supremacy is the state or condition of being Superior to all others in authority, power or status.

49.   Subdue: To gain control of (a violent or dangerous person or group) by using force, punishment. E.g. the troops were finally able to *subdue* the rebel forces after many days of fighting.
- To get control of (something, such as a strong emotion). She struggled to *subdue* her fears.

50.   Toxic: Containing poisonous substances (poisonous). A *toxic* substance/compound. E.g. the fumes from that chemical are highly *toxic*. Sometimes used figuratively a *toxic* (very unpleasant) work environment, relationship or emotion.

51.   Uterus: (Technical) womb; a hollow muscular organ in the pelvic cavity of female mammals, in which the embryo is nourished and develops before birth.
- Organ similar to mammalian womb; a structure in some animals that is similar to the mammalian womb, in which eggs or young develop.

52.   Vow: A serious promise to do something or to behave in a certain way
- The monks take a *vow* of silence/chastity/poverty.
- marriage/wedding *vows*
- The bride and groom exchanged *vows*.
- The mayor made a *vow* to reduce crime.

53.   Wedlock: Married state; the state of being married.

54.   Witchcraft: magical things that are done by witches. The use of magical powers obtained especially from evil spirits. E.g. the villagers blamed their problems on *witchcraft (sorcery)*

55.   Womanhood: The state or condition of being an adult woman and no longer a girl. A young girl on the verge of *womanhood.*

56. **Feminism:** The belief that men and women should have equal rights and opportunities. Or; organized activity in support of women's rights and interests

57. **Yokes:** Bar or frame that is attached to the heads or necks of two work animals (such as oxen) so that they can pull a plow or heavy load.

• Something that causes people to be treated cruelly and unfairly especially taking away their freedom.

God Bless You!

ABOUT THE AUTHOR

Janice N. Njie

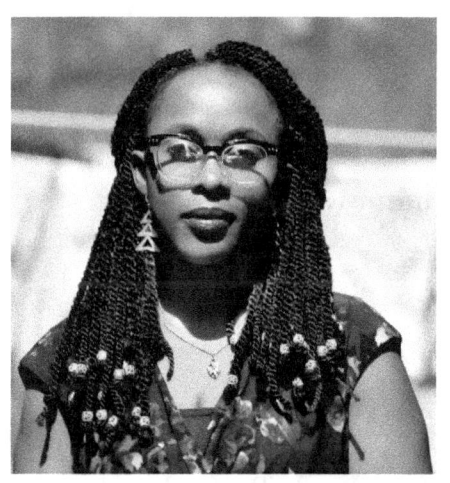

Janice lives with the unshakable belief that, as human beings, we were created spirit beings, blessed with a physical form and possessing a Soul. With the unique ability to communicate and interact with various spiritual realities.

Janice became a Christian after many years of experiencing different kinds of spiritual bonds with beings from other realities. For over two decades, Janice has preached the Gospel of Salvation, calling men to renounce Darkness by personal choice and deliberately surrender and follow the Lord Jesus Christ as their personal Lord and Savior.

For over two decades, Janice has preached the gospel amid her battles, struggles, challenges, and is a survivor of child sexual abuse, rape, domestic violence, spiritual/occultic manipulations from within, and outside church settings.

Janice is also a trained nurse, counselor, and holistic health practitioner. For many years, she has used her nursing career as a tool to reach the lost with the Good News of Salvation, deliverance, and Abundant Life in Christ Jesus.

Janice believes that as a nurse, her foremost calling, her gifts and talents are for healing, deliverance, and nurturing sick, broken, wounded lives, helping them to attain completion, fruitfulness, and abundant life through Christ Jesus.

Janice has written and published three books all of which are on Amazon.

You, Your Sexuality and God
Your Journey Towards Fertility
Broken Hedges

She is the mother of Victory Tijesunimi Njie-Atere.

CONTACT INFORMATION:

Email address: janicenjie73@gmail.com

Links:
https://spiritualityanddimensions.blogspot.com/
https://www.instagram.com/janiegracious/
https://web.facebook.com/groups/616579122310199